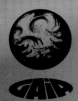

GAIA

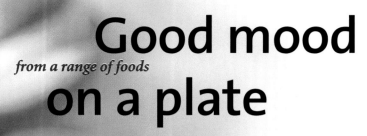

Good mood
from a range of foods
on a plate

FOOD & PSYCHE

We all feel low from time to time. Our moods – the close interplay between body and soul – are controlled biochemically by our brain. This is achieved by the release of chemical substances, neurotransmitters, that are manufactured at the speed of light when required – for example, serotonin and the endorphins. Certain substances in food are involved in the construction of these "happy messengers", and therefore have a direct effect on our performance, behaviour – and mood.

WORTH KNOWING

A good mood is linked to an overall feeling of relaxation and a rested body. If we are constantly under stress, we eventually start to feel unwell. So to keep your good mood, watch out for signals from your brain: don't work if you are feeling tired, but take a break. And don't rely on sugary "instant energy" drinks; they will only make you feel worse once the initial effects wear off.

THIS WILL DO YOU GOOD

✸ Absorb all the substances in your food that optimize the processes in your brain and that are used to manufacture neurotransmitters.

* Make sure you get enough sleep – 7 to 8 hours a night.
* Stay active – sport increases the serotonin level in your brain and stimulates the release of endorphins.

THESE WILL NOT....

* One of our worst enemies is a kind of fatty component: the so-called saturated fatty acids. They need lots of oxygen for burning, and so restrict the amount of oxygen that is transported to the brain. This makes us feel tired, lethargic, and can even lead to depression. There are lots of saturated fatty acids in foods such as fatty meat, bacon and processed meats, cheese, mayonnaise, and lots of sweets, pastries, and cakes.
* High alcohol consumption too has a negative effect on mood. It is also one of the worst enemies of the B complex – the vitamins that we need to manufacture our happy little messengers. However, small amounts of alcohol can sometimes have a beneficial effect on our moods.

FOOD FOR THE BRAIN

Our brain controls all the processes in our body, and it needs the following to do so:
* plenty of oxygen

* enough energy in the form of glucose, the smallest of the carbohydrates. Best obtained from wholewheat bread, cereals and grains, potatoes, wheat, and fresh vegetables and fruit, which are rich in other nutrients as well as carbohydrates.
* polyunsaturated fatty acids that look after the protective layer around our nerve cells and transmit information as quickly as possible. These fatty acids are contained in cold-pressed vegetable oils, nuts and seeds, and fish such as mackerel, herring, tuna, and salmon.
* Amino acids, the smallest protein molecules, are needed for the manufacture of neurotransmitters and hormones. Good sources are fish, seafood, lean meat, eggs, milk and dairy products, cheese, cereals, and pulses.
* A balanced cocktail of vitamins, minerals, and trace elements. This is needed for the biomechanical processes – to ignite the spark. These vital ingredients are present in good quantities in fresh fruit and vegetables, cereal and dairy products, lean meat, fish, nuts, seeds, and herbs.

RECOMMENDATION: Use organic produce wherever possible. If you wish to avoid genetically modified (GM) foods, read any labels with care and select certified organic produce, as this is not produced from GM ingredients.

Substances for

feel better every day

a good mood

SUBSTANCES THAT MAKE YOU HAPPY

Neurotransmitters transport information from one nerve cell to another. They are substances made by the body from the food we eat and manufactured in the brain. The building blocks for these are usually amino acids, and vitamins, minerals, trace elements, or fatty acids are also often required. Of the more than 60 different types of neurotransmitters that have been recognized to date, the following will make you feel happy:

SEROTONIN

This substance is also known as the "happy hormone" because it is the main chemical that produces a feeling of happiness in us. If we have enough of it, we feel balanced and content. Serotonin promotes relaxation and wellbeing, and aids deep sleep. If the brain does not have enough, our mood rapidly sinks. A deficiency can even make us aggressive. This messenger is manufactured from the amino acid tryptophan found in food. The less fat and the more carbohydrates are available, the more serotonin is produced.

ACETYLCHOLINE

This neurotransmitter is a product of choline, one of the B complex vitamins. Its many tasks include the promotion of concentration, alertness, learning, and memory. It makes us mentally fit, optimistic, and relaxed. Medication and drugs can have a seriously detrimental effect on its construction and effect.

DOPAMINE

This neurotransmitter stimulates the heart, circulation, and metabolism. It can mobilize the body's energy sources. The result: we are active and emotionally balanced. Dopamine lends our thoughts wings, and an excess can make us fantasize. We find ourselves daydreaming. However, a serious deficiency can leave us feeling listless, unmotivated, and emotionally empty.

NORADRENALINE

Along with serotonin, this is one of the main "happy hormones". Noradrenaline, produced by the body under stress, stimulates the brain, and promotes perception, motivation, and energy. It is also an anti-depressant. The latest research shows that not only does noradrenaline help us to concentrate in stressful situations, but it can also make us feel optimistic and euphoric - so stress obviously has a positive side! This substance also allows us to recall pleasure and strong emotions clearly and vividly. Noradrenaline is made from the amino acid phenylalanine.

ENDORPHINS AND NEUROPEPTIDES

The term endorphins refers to a group of the brain's own substances that act like drugs, either medicinal or social. They can reduce pain, and give rise to feelings of wellbeing and even euphoria. When our endorphin level rises, it provides a balanced psyche. Serotonin activates the endorphins; noradrenaline prevents this highly sensitive substance from breaking down too soon. Neuropeptides excite us, and so they control our emotions, our sexual and eating behaviour.

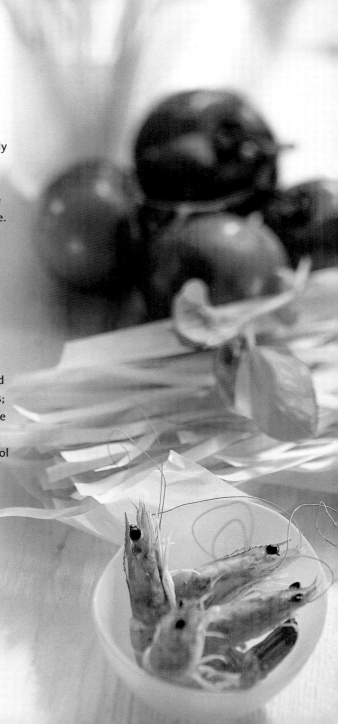

These foods

and they're stimulating and revitalizing

lift our mood

EAT WELL
AND BE HAPPY

Among the ingredients that our food is made from is a handful of substances that reinforce and increase the positive effects of the neurotransmitters. These include:

* About 30,000 different bioactive food components found in plants such as the natural colourings, aromas, and flavours that are present in substantial amounts in fresh fruit and vegetables. They play an important role in making sure ours is a healthy, vital organism.

* Spices: many of these are a tonic for the soul. Saffron, for example, helps to increase a feeling of joie de vivre. Nutmeg and cinnamon lift our mood. The sweet spices of vanilla release endorphins that lend us a feeling of wellbeing.

* Capsaicin: this substance provides the spicy heat in paprika and chilli. It also releases endorphins.

* Sinigrin: found in mustard and cruciferous vegetables such as Brussels sprouts, they can stimulate alertness and activity, and so increase a feeling of happiness.

* Analeptic amines are made from building blocks in oat protein, and help to release dopamine, which in turn is a precursor of serotonin. Analeptic amines not only promote concentration and performance; oats also lift the mood

* Caffeine: volunteers who have taken part in various studies admit that coffee (2 cups a day) left them feeling clearer, more confident, and more energetic. Caffeine probably supports the effects of the performance-enhancing hormones dopamine and noradrenaline. However, an excess has the opposite effect, and will make us feel shaky and on edge.

* The cocoa in chocolate contains several highly effective substances that reduce frustration and emotional problems (especially those of a romantic nature!), and lift our spirits. Theobromine, for example, stimulates the central nervous system, and phenylethylamine increases serotonin levels and our mood.

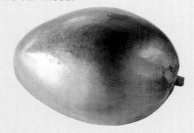

NEURO-TRANSMITTER	HELPS WITH	DERIVED FROM
Serotonin	Mood swings, craving for sweet food, unease, irritability, slight feelings of fear, problems falling asleep	Pasta, rice, potatoes, whole cereals, wholewheat bread, nuts, dates, figs, bananas, pineapple, confectionery, pulses, tofu, red vegetables, horseradish, fennel, dairy products, cheese, seafood, lean meat, poultry
Acetylcholine	Poor concentration, learning and memory, tenseness	Liver, egg yolks, cheese, oats, soy, lecithin, pulses, whole cereals, wholewheat bread, nuts, wheat germ, sesame seeds, yeast
Dopamine	Poor concentration, lack of motivation	Milk and dairy products, cheese, eggs, potatoes, rice, pasta, poultry, meat, fish, seafood
Noradrenaline	Psychological stress, poor sleep, tendency to depression, poor concentration, lack of motivation	Milk and dairy products, fish, seafood, eggs, poultry, meat, whole grains, pulses, red vegetables, spinach, apples, pineapple, nuts, chocolate
Endorphins and neuropeptides	Stress, pressure, mood swings, lethargy, depression	Fish, meat, poultry, dairy products, whole grains, pasta, wholewheat honey, bananas, dried fruit, chocolate and other confectionery

Power

the way to happiness

week

LIFT YOUR MOOD

Here's something you can do to help yourself when you are feeling sad, tired, and lethargic: treat yourself to 7 days of the best good mood foods. The recipes are healthy and uncomplicated to prepare, too. All in all, this week will harmonize your psyche, release positive energy, and help to make you happy.

THE PLAN

You will find suggestions for breakfast, lunch, and an evening meal for each day of the week. Of course, you can swap the meals if you want to, because all of the recipes in this book contain the "power foods" you need to feel more balanced and energetic. People who work away from home and are unable to cook 2 meals a day can choose an evening meal. You can also take the 2 sandwiches from the chapter on breakfasts (page 16) for your lunch break. The best choice is wholewheat bread with (not too fatty) cheese or Mozzarella with papaya and basil (page 27). Also good is fresh fruit, such as apples, pears, berries, bananas, figs, or pineapple, which you can combine with some yoghurt or with quark and eat when you are at work.

NATURAL ACTIVE SUBSTANCES

This is how foods can affect your particular needs:

* Performance and concentration need protein-rich foods such as milk and dairy products, fish, seafood, and lean meat. However, nuts, pulses, and wheat germ are also good.

* Stimulating substances are present in saffron, nutmeg, ginger, pepper, cinnamon, vanilla, peppermint, basil, and parsley.

* Wheat germ, oats, millet, rice, wholewheat bread, and almonds are very good for the nerves, as are liver and lean pork.

* Beat stress with milk and dairy products, eggs, cheese, fish, lean meat, whole foods, potatoes, vegetables, fruit, nuts, and sesame seeds.

THE PLAN

Monday

* Kefir muesli with strawberries
* Tomato drink with basil * Courgette rosti with smoked salmon strips
* Waldorf salad with pineapple

Tuesday

* Turkey breast sandwich
* Halibut with a rice and vegetable crust
* Tex-mex roll with avocado * Apricot quark gratin

Wednesday

* Berry and walnut yoghurt
* Mango lassi with maple syrup * Vegetable curry with peanuts
* Sweetcorn fritters with shrimps

Thursday

* Scrambled eggs with Cheddar; wholewheat bread
* Stuffed potatoes; mixed leaf salad
* Creamy saffron soup * Pineapple and papaya salad

Friday

* Buckthorn quark with grapes
* Oven-baked tuna; plain boiled rice
* Couscous salad with red vegetables

Saturday

* Gorgonzola sandwich
* Vegetable casserole with millet * Chocolate mousse
* Beetroot and orange salad; five-grain bread

Sunday

* Smoked salmon mousse with wholewheat baguette
* Chilli chicken with mango * Refreshing lemon kefir drink
* Red lentil and rocket salad

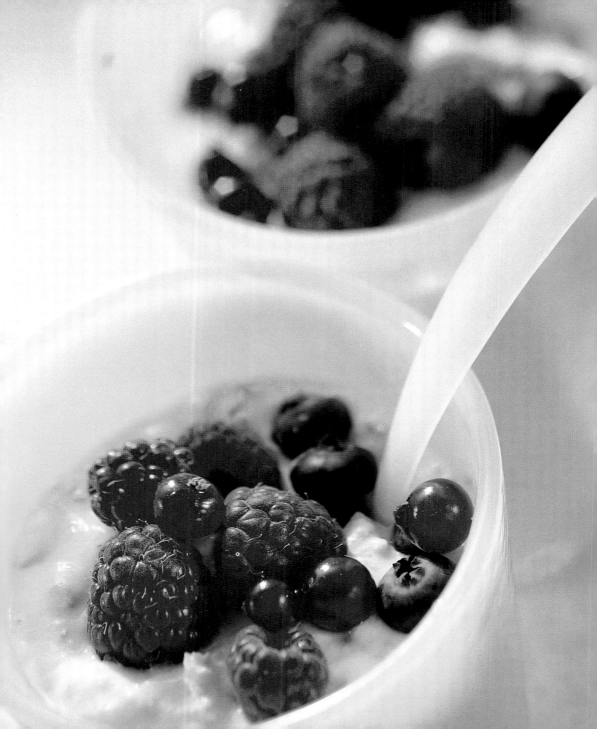

Walnut

with golden-yellow

berry

toasted oats

yoghurt

Serves 2: • 4 tbsp oatmeal • 2 tbsp walnut halves • 300 g (10 oz) yoghurt

(1.5% fat) • 1–2 tsp acacia honey • 100 g (3 ¹/₂ oz) mixed berries

Dry-fry the oatmeal in a small nonstick frying pan until golden. Chop the walnuts. Combine the nuts and the oatmeal with the yoghurt, and sweeten with honey.

Pour the nut yoghurt into tall glasses. Rinse the berries and use to decorate the yoghurt.

PER PORTION: 250 kcal • 9 g protein • 13 g fat • 24 g carbohydrate

Kefir muesli

naturally sweetened with maple syrup

with strawberries

Serves 2: • 1 banana • 100 g (3 ¹/₂ oz) strawberries • 4 tbsp unsweetened muesli • 2 tbsp wheat germ • 200 g (7 oz) kefir (1.5% fat) or probiotic yoghurt drink • 2 tsp maple syrup • 1 sprig of lemon balm

Peel and slice the banana. Wash, hull, and quarter the strawberries. Arrange the fruit on one half of a plate. Combine the muesli and the wheat germ, and arrange beside the fruit. Divide the kefir between the fruit and the muesli, and sprinkle over the maple syrup. Decorate with lemon balm.

PER PORTION: 190 kcal • 7 g protein • 3 g fat • 42 g carbohydrate

Buckthorn quark

with plenty of vitamin C

with grapes

Serves 2: • 200 g (7 oz) green and black grapes • 200 g (7 oz) prepared quark (1.5% fat) • 4 tbsp buckthorn syrup • ¹/₂ tsp vanilla extract • 2 tbsp ground hazelnuts • 1 tbsp lemon juice

Wash the grapes. Pull from the stalks and cut in half lengthwise. Remove the seeds if preferred. Combine the quark with the buckthorn syrup, vanilla extract, and hazelnuts, and season with lemon juice. Layer two-thirds of the grapes and the quark mixture in small glass dishes. Top with the remaining grapes.

PER PORTION: 245 kcal • 16 g protein • 3 g fat • 27 g carbohydrate

Scrambled eggs
on tasty rye bread
with Cheddar

Lightly beat together the eggs with the milk, a little pepper, and some salt until the mixture is smooth but not fluffy. Melt the butter in a nonstick pan over a medium heat.

Pour in the eggs and leave to set slightly over a low heat. Using a palette knife, gently push the outside to the centre from time to time.

Wash the bell pepper, then trim, and finely chop.

Sprinkle over the scrambled eggs with the Cheddar and allow the cheese to melt. The eggs are ready when set, but still creamy and shiny.

Arrange the scrambled eggs on the bread, and serve warm.

Serves 2:

3 eggs

4 tbsp milk

white pepper

salt

1 tbsp butter

$1/2$ small red bell pepper

4 tbsp coarsely grated Cheddar

4 slices of wholewheat bread

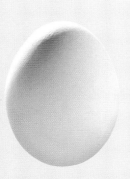

Hens' eggs

They are one of the most nutritious foods. Their proportion of fat-soluble vitamins and vitamins B_2, B_{12}, and folic acid is unusually high. Eggs contain a good amount of lecithin, which is considered essential for the brain and nerves. The amino acid tryptophan plays a key role in the manufacture of the "happy hormone" serotonin.

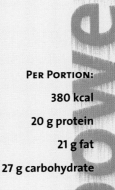

PER PORTION:

380 kcal

20 g protein

21 g fat

27 g carbohydrate

power

Smoked salmon
mousse

for Sundays and special occasions

Serves 2:
75 g (scant 3 oz) smoked salmon
1 tbsp olive oil
1 tbsp soft butter
30 g (1 oz) low-fat quark
salt
pepper
1–2 tbsp lemon juice
1/2 bunch of chives
150 g (5 oz) salmon fillet
4 slices of multi-grain bread

Cut the smoked salmon into large pieces. Then place the salmon, olive oil, butter, quark, a little salt, pepper, and 1 tablespoon of lemon juice in a blender, and blend until smooth.

Wash the chives, shake dry, and cut into short lengths. Chop the salmon fillet into small pieces and stir into the mousse with the chives. Season with salt, pepper, and the remaining lemon juice. Place in the refrigerator until ready to serve. Serve for breakfast with warm, crispy multi-grain toast.

Omega-3 fatty acids for the brain

Salmon contains more Omega-3 fatty acids than almost any other variety of fish. They protect the nerve cells and facilitate the flow of information. Its amino acids and vitamins are needed for the construction of a number of hormones that prevent negative emotions, and can even increase our sensual perception. So fish is definitely good for the mind and the body!

PRO PORTION:

375 kcal

32 g protein

19 g fat

18 g carbohydrate

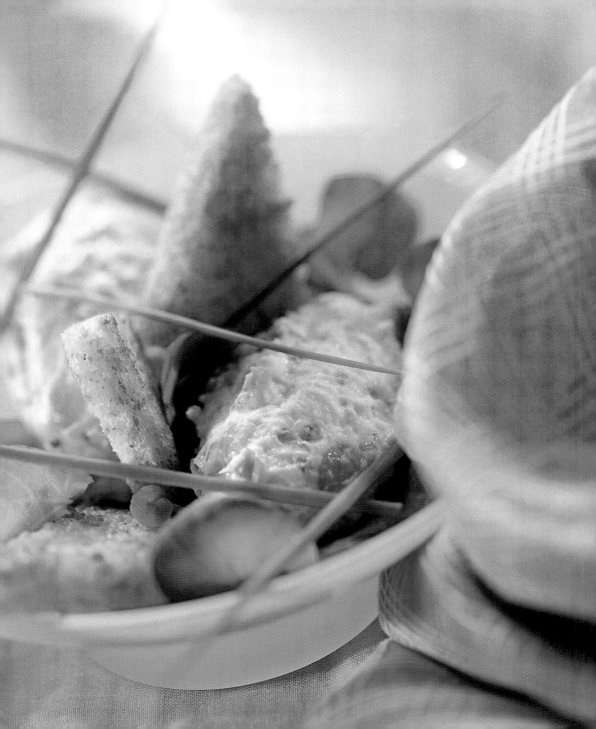

Turkey breast

light, nutritious, and good for a packed lunch

sandwich

Serves 2: • 2 wholewheat bread rolls • 50 g (scant 2 oz) cucumber • $\frac{1}{2}$ red bell pepper • 50 g (scant 2 oz) buttermilk cheese (8% fat) • black pepper • 4 leaves rocket (arugula) • 50 g (scant 2 oz) cold turkey breast

Halve the bread rolls lengthwise. Wash the cucumber and cut into slices. Halve the bell pepper. Wash, trim, and chop finely. Combine with the cheese and season with pepper. Spread over the bread rolls. Place 2 leaves of rocket, the sliced cucumber, and the turkey breast on the bottom halves of the rolls. Top with the other half.

PER PORTION: 275 kcal • 14 g protein • 6 g fat • 41 g carbohydrate

Gorgonzola

with fresh figs and pistachios

sandwich

Serves 2: • 1 tbsp shelled pistachios • 2 long wholewheat bread rolls • 2 fresh, ripe figs • 100 g (3 $\frac{1}{2}$ oz) Gorgonzola • 4 leaves of lollo rosso

Coarsely chop the pistachios and dry-fry in a frying pan. Leave to cool. Cut the rolls into half lengthwise. Wash and pat dry the figs. Slice the figs and the Gorgonzola. Place the salad leaves, cheese, and figs on the bottom halves of the rolls, and sprinkle with the pistachios. Top with the other half.

PER PORTION: 400 kcal • 16 g protein • 19 g fat • 42 g carbohydrate

Ham tartare
with lots of bioactive substances
with vegetables

Drain the mixed pickles in a sieve, then chop as finely as possible. Wash and dry the apple, and cut into quarters. Remove the seeds and core, then finely chop the apple quarters. Remove the fatty rind from the ham, and chop the ham into small pieces. Combine the mixed pickles, chopped apple, and chopped ham in a bowl. Add the yoghurt and mustard, and stir. Season to taste with pepper. Divide the ham tartare between the slices of bread, cut each slice into half diagonally, and sprinkle over the chopped chives or cress.

Serves 2:
50 g (scant 2 oz) mixed pickles (ready bought)
1 small apple
100 g (3 ½ oz) cooked ham
2 tbsp yoghurt (1.5% fat)
¼ tsp mustard
white pepper
4 slices of dark wholewheat bread
1 tbsp chopped chives or cress

Pickles for a kick

Mixed pickles, vegetables preserved in vinegar, contain lactic acid bacteria, which have a beneficial effect on our metabolism. They protect us against harmful bacteria and fungus, so they help to protect us against infection and strengthen our immune system. This keeps the body healthy and fit.

PER PORTION:

370 kcal

20 g protein

11 g fat

47 g carbohydrate

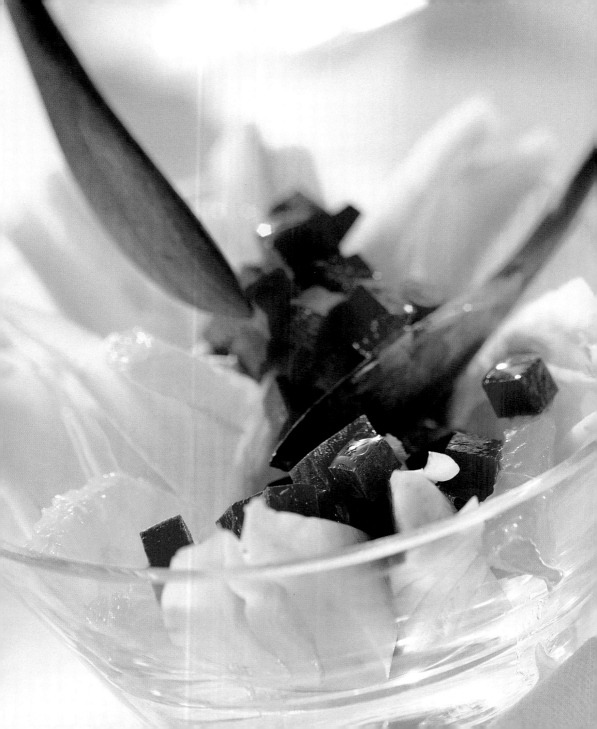

Beetroot and orange salad

full of serotonin and bioactive plant materials

Wash, peel, and dice the beetroot. Place in a pan with 75 ml (3 fl oz) water and the maple syrup. Cover with a lid and simmer gently for 8–10 minutes.

Remove from the heat and add the lemon juice and sherry. Cover and leave overnight in the refrigerator. Drain the beetroot. Peel the oranges, then halve and cut into thin slices, saving the juice. Reserve 2 tablespoons of the juice and add the rest to the beetroot. Wash and trim the fennel, then slice as thinly as possible.

Combine the reserved orange juice with a little salt, pepper, and oil, and sprinkle over the sliced fennel. Then arrange on plates with the sliced orange and the beetroot. Roughly chop the cashew nuts, and sprinkle over the salad.

Serves 2:
- 200 g (7 oz) small beetroot
- 1 tbsp maple syrup
- 2 tbsp lemon juice
- 2 tbsp cream sherry
- 2 small oranges
- 1 small fennel (150 g/5 oz)
- salt
- white pepper
- 1 tbsp olive oil
- 2 tbsp cashew nuts

PER PORTION: 250 kcal • 6 g protein • 11 g fat • 28 g carbohydrate

Waldorf salad
refreshing and full of vitamins
with pineapple

Serves 2:
3 tbsp walnuts
100 g (3 ¹/₂ oz) sticks of celery
100 g (3 ¹/₂ oz) celeriac
2 tbsp lemon juice
2 red-skinned apples
2 tbsp yoghurt-based salad dressing (30% fat)
2 tbsp cream or milk
white pepper
100 g (3 ¹/₂ oz) fresh pineapple

Roughly chop 2 tablespoons of the walnuts. Wash, trim, and finely chop the sticks of celery. Finely chop the tender green shoots. Wash, peel, and grate or finely chop the celeriac, and mix well with the lemon juice.

Wash, dry, and quarter the apples. Remove the cores and finely chop the apple quarters. Add to the grated or chopped celeriac. Blend the salad dressing with the cream or milk, and season with a little pepper. Combine with the apple and celeriac mixture, walnuts, and chopped celery. Cover and chill for 1 hour. Chop the pineapple and add to the Waldorf salad. Garnish with the remaining walnuts, and serve.

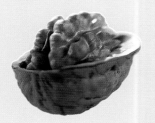

Walnuts

These aromatic nuts are simply bursting with nutrition: amino acids, vitamins, minerals, and lots of unsaturated fatty acids. This "power bomb" revitalizes the grey cells, banishes tiredness and stress, and makes us fit and active. Beneficial to the mood and wellbeing.

PER PORTION:

325 Kcal

6 g protein

21 g fat

26 g carbohydrate

Couscous salad
with lots of serotonin
with red vegetables

Peel and finely chop the carrot, onion, and garlic. Heat the oil in a pan and sauté the carrot, onion, and garlic. Pour over the stock, cover, and simmer gently for 2 minutes. Stir in the couscous, bring to a boil, and remove from the heat. Leave to stand according to the packet instructions. Drain the couscous and leave to cool.

Wash, trim, and finely chop the tomatoes and bell pepper. Wash and pat dry the salad, and tear into pieces.

Combine the vinegar, salt, pepper, and olive oil. Use to dress the vegetables and the salad leaves. Season the couscous with lemon juice, salt, and pepper. Arrange on plates with the vegetables, salad, and basil leaves.

Serves 2:

1 carrot
1 small red onion
1 clove of garlic
2 tsp oil
150 ml (5 fl oz) vegetable stock
200 g (7 oz) couscous
2 tomatoes
1 small red bell pepper
4 leaves of lollo rosso
3 tbsp white wine vinegar
salt, black pepper
1 tbsp cold-pressed olive oil
3–4 tbsp lemon juice
fresh basil leaves

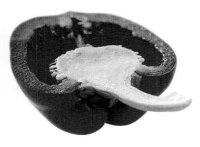

Red vegetables

The colours of vegetable influence the psyche just as much as their vital constituents do. Red symbolizes warmth, strength, and life energy. Vegetables such as tomatoes, red bell peppers, beetroot, carrots, kidney beans, and red cabbage create optimism and a positive attitude to life.

PER PORTION:

500 kcal

13 g protein

14 g fat

79 g carbohydrate

Red lentil and
with warm goat's cheese
rocket salad

Heat the olive oil in a pan and briefly sauté the rosemary. Add the lentils and stock, and cover with a lid. Simmer gently for 10 minutes.

Serves 2:
2 tbsp olive oil
2 tsp fresh rosemary
100 g (3 ½ oz) red lentils
200 ml (7 fl oz) vegetable stock
2 spring onions (scallions)
1 bunch of rocket (arugula)
(50 g/scant 2 oz)
2 tbsp white wine vinegar
salt
white pepper
1 tbsp sunflower oil
1 clove of garlic
2 small round goat's cheeses
(50 g/scant 2 oz each)

Meanwhile, wash and trim the spring onions, and cut into thin rings. Trim, pick over, and wash the rocket. Shake dry and tear any large leaves. Drain the lentils in a sieve. Combine the vinegar, salt, pepper, and sunflower oil, and stir 2 tablespoons into the lentils. Peel and crush the garlic, and add to the lentils. Season to taste with salt and pepper.

Cut across (but not through) each side of the goat's cheese several times to make a star shape. Heat in a nonstick pan without oil until just turning colour. Add the spring onions, rocket, and the remaining marinade to the lentil salad, and arrange on plates with the goat's cheese.

Lentils for a lift

Like peas and beans, red lentils are a pulse, and contain excellent amounts of minerals, and plenty of vitamin B1, the power pack for brain and muscles. They also contain a huge amount of plant protein and carbohydrate, and tryptophan, from which serotonin is made, is present in abundance.

PER PORTION:

395 kcal

23 g protein

20 g fat

31 g carbohydrate

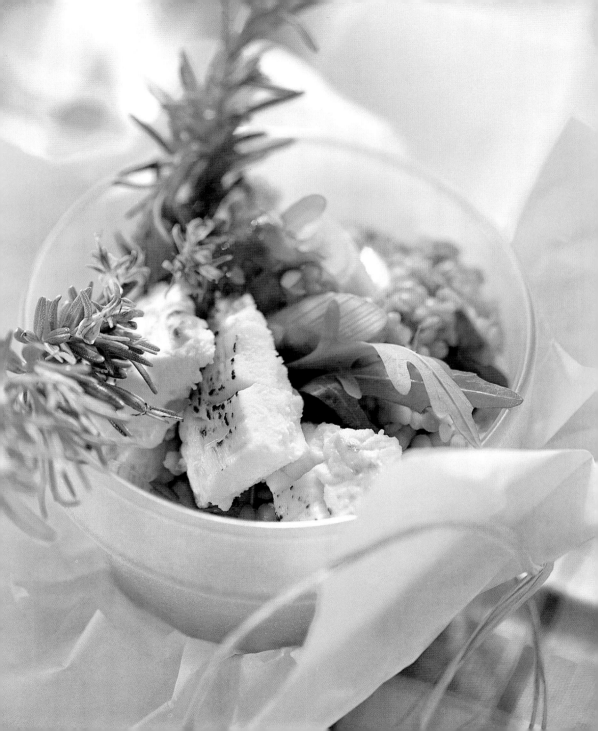

Creamy

with leeks and toasted almonds

saffron soup

Toast the bread and cut into small pieces. Peel and finely chop the shallot and garlic. Trim and wash the leek, and cut into thin rings. Heat the oil in a pan and sauté the leek, garlic, and shallot for 4 minutes. Set aside 1 generous tablespoon of the vegetables. Add the bread cubes and the saffron to the remaining vegetables. Pour over the stock and bring to a boil. Cover with a lid and simmer gently for 30 minutes. Stir the cream into the soup and season with salt and pepper. Dry-fry the almond flakes in a nonstick frying pan until golden. Divide the saffron soup between 2 bowls. Sprinkle with the reserved vegetables and the toasted almonds, and serve.

Serves 2:
40 g (1 ¹/₂ oz) wholewheat toast
1 shallot
1 small clove of garlic
1 tender leek (100 g/3 ¹/₂ oz)
1 tbsp olive oil
¹/₄ tsp ground saffron
600 ml (20 fl oz) vegetable stock
3 tbsp cream
salt
white pepper
1 tbsp almond flakes

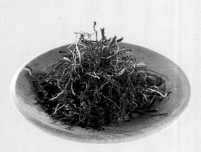

Saffron

Saffron is the most expensive spice in the world. The stigmas of a Mediterranean crocus are picked by hand, then dried. Not only does saffron add a delightful yellow colour and slightly bitter-sweet flavour, its bioactive substances and essential oils are balm for the soul.
Saffron has long been valued for its aphrodisiac qualities.

PRO PORTION:

205 kcal

4 g protein

13 g fat

16 g carbohydrate

power

Yoghurt soup

with flat sesame cakes

with red bell pepper

Cut the bell pepper into quarters, remove the white skin and the seeds, and wash. Cut the quarters widthwise into thin strips. Wash, trim, and diagonally slice the scallions. Peel and finely chop the garlic.

Combine the yoghurt, meat stock, and the egg in a pan. Stirring continuously over a medium heat, bring almost to a boil. Remove from the heat and season with salt and pepper. Stir occasionally.

Heat the olive oil in a small frying pan, and sauté half the sliced bell pepper, the spring onions, and the garlic for 3 minutes. Wash and shake dry the mint. Chop finely, reserving a few leaves as garnish. Purée the soup with a stick blender and divide between 2 bowls. Combine the vegetables and the chopped mint, and sprinkle over the yoghurt soup. Garnish with the reserved mint leaves.

Serves 2:

1 red bell pepper
2 spring onions (scallions)
1 clove of garlic
250 g (9 oz) whole milk yoghurt
200 ml (7 fl oz) meat stock (home-made is best)
1 egg
salt
white pepper
3 sprigs of fresh mint

power

PER PORTION: 180 kcal • 9 g protein • 12 g fat • 9 g carbohydrate

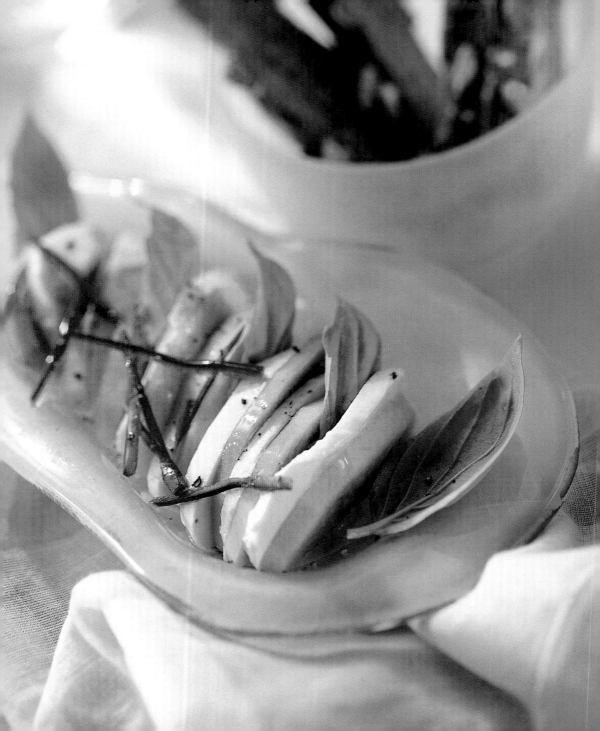

Mozzarella

seasoned with basil and chilli oil

with papaya

Cut open the chilli, and remove the seeds and pith. Wash, trim, and slice as thinly as possible. Combine with the oil and the salt in a bowl, and leave to stand for about 20 minutes.

Halve the whole Mozzarella ball and cut all 3 halves into very thin slices. Peel the papaya, cut in half lengthwise, and scoop out the seeds with a spoon. Slice the papaya halves widthwise. Wash the basil if required and shake dry. Remove the stalks.

Arrange the sliced Mozzarella, papaya, and basil on 2 plates, and sprinkle over the chilli oil. Serve with the sunflower seed rolls.

Serves 2:

1 small red chilli pod

3 tbsp soy or rapeseed oil (canola)

pinch of salt

1 ¹/₂ balls Mozzarella

3 sprigs of basil

2 sunflower seed bread rolls

Exotic power fruit

Papaya contains beta-carotene, which protects the nerve cells the production of free radicals very active molecules that can attack cells and tissues. Papain, an enzyme, stimulates the metabolism, boosts our energy – and our mood!

PER PORTION:

450 kcal

23 g protein

39 g fat

4 g carbohydrate

Mango lassi

Indian vitamin boost

with maple syrup

For 2 drinks: • 300 g (10 oz) mild yoghurt (1.5% fat) • 100 ml (3 ¹/₂ fl oz) mineral water • 4 tbsp mango purée, unsweetened • 3 tbsp lemon juice • 2–3 tbsp maple syrup • mint leaves

Whisk together the yoghurt, mineral water, mango, and lemon juice, either with a hand whisk or in an electric mixer, until the surface becomes frothy. Sweeten with maple syrup and pour into 2 tall glasses. Decorate with the mint leaves.

PER DRINK: 165 kcal • 5 g protein • 3 g fat • 30 g carbohydrate

Fruit mix

try it with fresh ginger

with wheat germ

For 2 drinks: • 1 slice of honey melon (150 g/5 oz) • ¹/₂ a banana • juice of 4 oranges • 2 tbsp wheat germ (from healthfood stores) • ¹/₄ tsp ground ginger

Peel the melon and remove the seeds. Chop into small pieces. Peel and slice the banana. Combine the fruit with the orange juice, wheat germ, and ginger in a tall mixer goblet, and purée with a stick blender. Pour into 2 large glasses and drink through thick straws.

PER DRINK: 155 kcal • 4 g protein • 1 g fat • 31 g carbohydrate

Refreshing
a power drink that boosts the brain
citrus kefir drink

For 2 drinks: • 250 g (9 oz) kefir (1.5% fat) (probiotic yoghurt drink) • 200 ml (7 fl oz) freshly squeezed orange juice • juice of 1 lime • 2 tbsp lecithin granules (from healthfood stores) • 1 tbsp runny honey • 1/4 tsp powdered vanilla

Combine the kefir, the orange and lime juices, the lecithin granules, and two-thirds of the honey in a tall mixer goblet and mix together until smooth. Sweeten with the remaining honey. Pour into 2 glasses and sprinkle with the vanilla.

PER DRINK: 280 kcal • 5 g protein • 17 g fat • 23 g carbohydrate

Tomato drink
serve chilled
with basil

For 2 drinks: • 4 ripe beef tomatoes • 100 g (3 1/2 oz) curds • 1 tbsp basil leaves • pinch of sugar • few drops of Tabasco

Wash and chop the tomatoes, removing the stalks. Combine the tomatoes, curds, basil, and sugar in a tall mixer goblet, and purée well with a stick blender. Season with the Tabasco, adding a drop at a time. Pour into 2 glasses.

PER DRINK: 70 kcal • 4 g protein • 2 g fat • 8 g carbohydrate

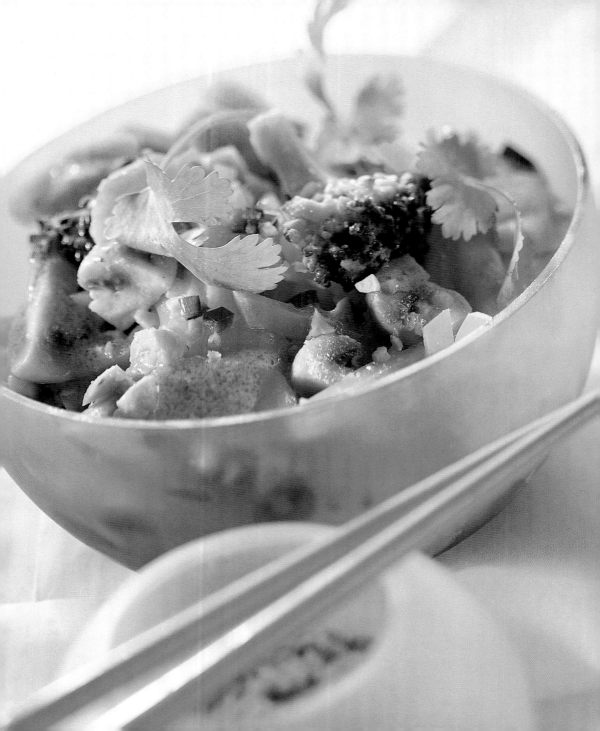

Vegetable curry

spiced up with chilli and fresh ginger

with peanuts

Cook the rice according to the packet instructions. Peel and finely chop the ginger, garlic, and shallots. Cut open the chilli pods. Wash and trim, then slice thinly. Wash and trim the broccoli, and divide into florets. Wash and trim the carrots, and slice diagonally. Halve the bell pepper and remove the seeds and pith. Wash the halves and slice. Wipe the mushrooms, then cut into quarters.

Heat the oil in a wok or a large frying pan. Stir-fry the ginger, garlic, shallots, and chilli pods briefly, then add the curry paste and stir briefly. Gradually add the coconut milk. Add the broccoli and carrots, and stir-fry for about 3 minutes. Add the remaining vegetables and continue to cook until everything is just *al dente*. Season to taste with salt and lemon juice.

Roughly chop the peanuts and sprinkle over the curry with the coriander leaves. Arrange on plates with the rice.

Serves 2:
125 g (4 oz) Basmati rice
15 g (1/2 oz) ginger
1 clove of garlic
2 shallots
1–2 chilli pods
200 g (7 oz) broccoli
2 carrots
1 yellow bell pepper
100 g (3 1/2 oz) mushrooms
1 tbsp oil
2 tsp red curry paste
300 ml (10 fl oz) unsweetened coconut milk
salt
1–2 tsp lemon juice
2 tbsp salted peanuts
2 tbsp coriander leaves (cilantro)

power

PER PORTION: 385 kcal • 14 g protein • 12 g fat • 60 g carbohydrate

Sweetcorn fritters

excellent with a mixed salad

with shrimps

Drain the corn in a strainer, then purée with 1 tablespoon of the cottage cheese with a stick blender. Drain the remaining cottage cheese.

Serves 2:
100 g (3 ½ oz) corn (canned)
50 g (scant 2 oz) cottage cheese
50 g (scant 2 oz) shrimps
1 small carrot
1 small clove of garlic
1 egg yolk
2 tbsp grated coconut
salt
black pepper
1 tbsp semolina or flour
2–3 tbsp oil
1 tbsp chopped parsley

Pat the shrimps dry with paper towels and chop them roughly. Wash, peel, and finely grate the carrot. Combine the shrimps and the grated carrot with the corn. Peel the garlic and crush onto the carrot and corn mixture. Stir in the egg yolk, grated coconut, salt, pepper, and semolina or flour.

Heat the oil in a frying pan. Fry a total of 6 fritters over a medium heat for about 3 minutes on each side. Drain on paper towels.

Combine the remaining cottage cheese with the parsley. Arrange the fritters on plates, spoon a dollop of cottage cheese in the centre of each one, and serve immediately while hot.

power

PER PORTION: 300 kcal • 13 g protein • 21 g fat • 16 g carbohydrate

Spaghetti with
interesting with Parma ham and capers
broccoli cream

Chop half of the pistachio nuts roughly, and the other half finely. Drain the capers well. Wash and trim the broccoli. Divide into small florets and blanch in boiling salted water for 3 minutes. Drain, rinse under running cold water, and drain well in a strainer.

Bring plenty of salted water to a boil and cook the spaghetti according to the packet instruction. Meanwhile, peel and finely chop the shallot. Heat the oil in a pan, and sauté the shallot. Add half the broccoli, the vegetable stock, the quark, and the finely chopped pistachios. Purée everything with a stick blender until creamy. Season with salt, pepper, and lemon juice. Cut the ham into thick strips. Heat the remaining broccoli florets in the sauce. Quickly drain the spaghetti, and arrange on 2 plates with the vegetable purée, and the sliced ham. Sprinkle with the capers and the roughly chopped pistachios.

Serves 2:
2 tbsp pistachio nuts
1–2 tbsp small capers
300 g (10 oz) broccoli
salt
200 g (7 oz) spaghetti
1 shallot
1 tbsp oil
150 ml (5 fl oz) vegetable stock
100 g (3 ½ oz) quark with herbs (0.2% fat)
black pepper
2 tsp lemon juice
50 g (scant 2 oz) Parma ham

PER PORTION: 590 kcal • 28 g protein • 17 g fat • 83 g carbohydrate

Tex-mex roll

for an energy boost

with avocado

Wash the tomato, remove the stalk, then dice. Trim, wash, and finely chop the bell pepper and celery. Peel the avocado, cut in half lengthwise, and remove the pit. Finely chop one half, and purée the other with 1 tablespoon of lemon juice and the yoghurt. Roughly combine the puréed and the chopped avocado, chopped vegetables, and 1 ¹/₂ tablespoons of the herbs. Season with salt, sambal oelek, and the remaining lemon juice. Spread the filling over the tortillas, then roll and chill until ready to serve. Slice in half diagonally to arrange, and garnish with the remaining herbs.

Serves 2:
1 tomato
¹/₂ yellow bell pepper
¹/₂ stick of celery
1 small ripe avocado
1–2 tbsp lemon juice
1 tbsp yoghurt
2 tbsp chopped coriander (cilantro)
or parsley leaves
salt
¹/₄ tsp sambal oelek finely chopped
(chilli)
2 pre-cooked soft tortillas (ready
made; 16 cm/5 ¹/₂ inch diameter)

Solo or not

The Tex-mex roll can either be eaten as a vegetarian meal with a large salad of mixed leaves, or served as an unusual accompaniment to grilled meat such as chicken drumsticks, cutlets, or steak.

PER PORTION:

220 kcal

7 g protein

9 g fat

29 g carbohydrate

power

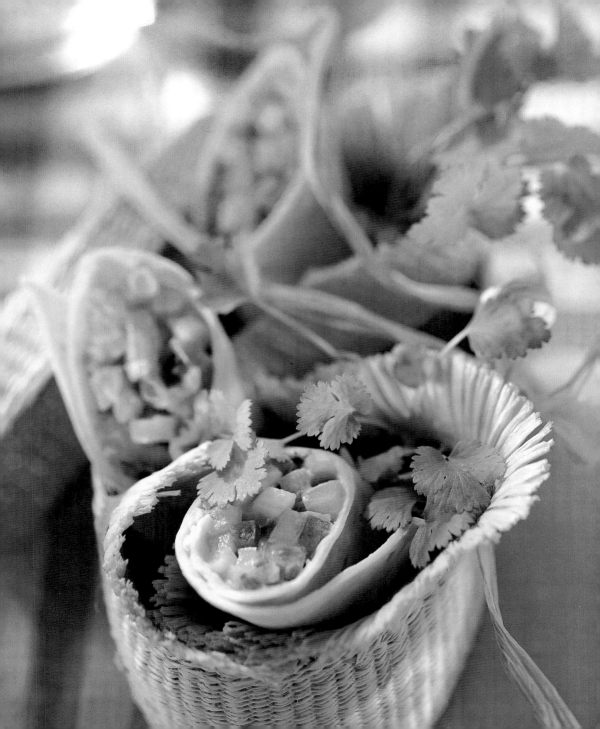

Vegetable casserole
lots of serotonin and iron for more elan
with millet

Bring the millet to a boil in 150 ml (5 fl oz) of the vegetable stock. Cover, turn off the heat, and leave to absorb for about 20 minutes. Meanwhile, wash and peel the carrots and kohlrabi. Slice the carrots and dice the kohlrabi. Peel and finely chop the onion.

Heat the oil in a pan and sauté the carrots, kohlrabi, and onion. Add the remaining stock, mustard, bay leaf, a little salt, and pepper. Bring to a boil, cover, and simmer gently for 10 minutes.

Wash and pick over the spinach. Remove any coarse stalks and tear the leaves into pieces. Wash the tomatoes and remove the stalks, then dice them. Simmer both with the peas for another 10 minutes. Peel the garlic, crush, and add to the vegetables. Stir in the herbs and the millet. Season with salt and pepper, and serve immediately.

Serves 2:
75 g (scant 3 oz) millet
1 litre (35 fl oz) vegetable stock
200 g (7 oz) carrots
1 kohlrabi
1 onion
2 tbsp olive oil
1–2 tsp hot mustard
1 bay leaf
salt
pepper
handful of spinach leaves
2 tomatoes
150 g (5 oz) frozen peas
1 clove of garlic
3 tbsp herbs (e.g. parsley or chives)

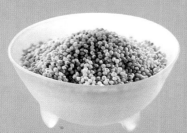

Millet
These tiny golden grains are full of important nutrients. They contain good amounts of iron, manganese, copper, magnesium, fluoride, silicic acid, B complex vitamins, and lecithin, so they are the ideal brain food. This power mix makes us feel awake, full of life, and happy.

PER PORTION:
430 kcal
12 g protein
15 g fat
60 g carbohydrate

Courgette rosti

for instant energy

with salmon strips

Using a balloon whisk, beat together the eggs, flour, salt, and thyme in a bowl. Cover and chill for 15 minutes in the refrigerator. Meanwhile, peel and finely chop the shallot. Wash and trim the courgettes, and grate roughly. Add the shallot, the grated courgettes, and the cream to the dough. Season with salt and pepper.

Heat the oil in a large frying pan over a medium heat. Prepare 6–8 rosti, frying for about 3 minutes on each side. Drain on paper towels.

Cut the gravadlax into wide strips, and arrange on plates with the courgette rosti. Combine the yoghurt and the lime juice, and sprinkle over the gravadlax.

Serves 2:
2 eggs
50 g (scant 2 oz) flour
salt
1 tsp dried thyme
1 shallot
250 g (9 oz) courgettes (zucchini)
2 tbsp cream
black pepper
2–3 tbsp oil
50 g (scant 2 oz) gravadlax (marinated salmon)
3 tbsp yoghurt (1.5% fat)
2–3 tbsp lime juice

power

PER PORTION: 420 kcal • 18 g protein • 24 g fat • 33 g carbohydrate

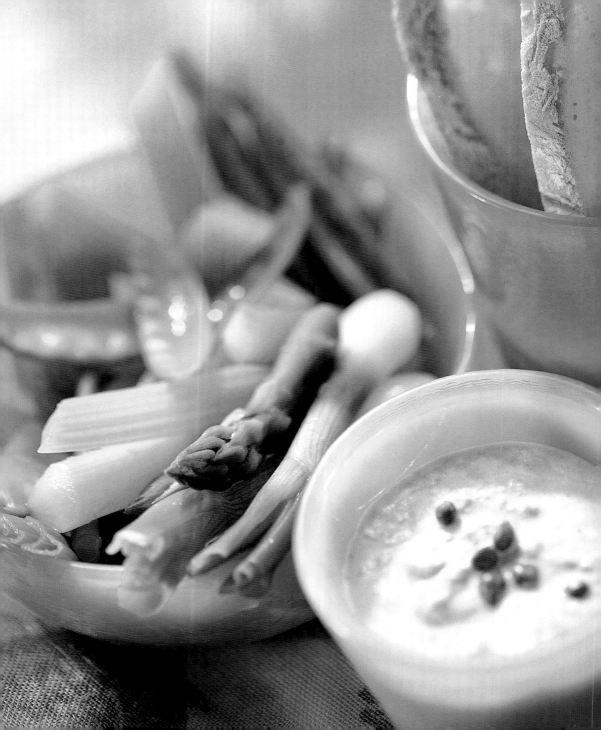

Green vegetables
with tuna sauce

with plenty of relaxing calcium and magnesium

Wash and trim the vegetables. Peel the lower third of the asparagus. Cut the courgettes lengthwise into quarters. Cut the asparagus, courgettes, celery, and spring onions into bean-length pieces.

Wash the lime under hot water, dry, and grate. Squeeze out the juice. Place the vegetables in a flat dish, season lightly with salt and pepper, and sprinkle over the lime rind. Wash the parsley, and reserve 3 stalks.

Pour 200 ml/7 fl oz of water into a wide pan, then add 1/2 teaspoon salt, the asparagus trimmings, and the parsley. Place the fish on a steam insert over the pan, then cover and steam the vegetables for about 10–12 minutes until *al dente*.

Drain the tuna, then purée thoroughly with the crème fraîche and 2 tablespoons of lime juice. Finely chop the remaining parsley and add to the sauce with the capers. Season the sauce and serve with the vegetables.

Serves 2:
800 g (1 3/4 lb) mixed
vegetables (e.g. green
asparagus, courgettes, celery,
beans, spring onions
(scallions), mange-tout)
1 lime
salt
white pepper
1/2 bunch of parsley
small can of tuna in
brine (80 g/3 oz)
1 tbsp crème fraîche
2 tsp small capers

Green vegetables for more vitality

Green is the colour of hope, it is said, and it means finding new hope. If you are feeling under the weather, treat yourself to something green. Either eat the vegetables raw, or cook them carefully to retain the maximum amount of vitamins and minerals. Green vegetables calm us down, relax us, and reduce aggression.

PER PORTION:
235 kcal
24 g protein
14 g fat
30 g carbohydrate

Stuffed
with spicy almond spinach
potatoes

Brush the potatoes thoroughly under running water. Leave them unpeeled and cook for 30 minutes. Meanwhile, wash and pick over the spinach, removing any thick stalks. Place the wet

Serves 2:
**3 firm potatoes (about
200–250 g/7–9 oz each)**
200 g (7 oz) leaf spinach
½ a courgette (zucchini)
1 onion
2 tbsp olive oil
1 egg
50 g (scant 2 oz) Gorgonzola
**30 g (1 oz) freshly ground
almonds**
2–3 tbsp whole milk yoghurt
salt
white pepper

spinach in a pan over a high heat until it has wilted. Drain well in a sieve and chop roughly. Wash and roughly grate the courgette. Peel, and chop the onion. Heat the oil, and sauté the onion and the grated zucchini for 2 minutes. Drain the potatoes, cut in half lengthwise, and scoop out some of the flesh. Mash the flesh and combine with the spinach, the onion/courgette mixture, egg, Gorgonzola, almonds, and yoghurt. Season to taste with salt and pepper, and divide between the potato halves. Place on a baking sheet and bake in the middle of the oven for about 15 minutes.

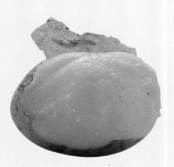

Potatoes

As well as plenty of vitamins, minerals, and fibre, potatoes contain a good supply of carbohydrate which helps to stimulate the production of seratonin, one of the major "happy hormones".

PER PORTION:

645 kcal

24 g protein

34 g fat

62 g carbohydrate

power

Potatoes with

with lots of revitalizing, exotic spices

tomato yoghurt

Combine the spices. To make the sauce, wash and halve the tomatoes. Remove the stalks and the seeds, and finely chop the flesh. Combine the yoghurt and the chopped tomatoes with a quarter of the mixed spices. Wash and shake dry the coriander or parsley, then pull the leaves from the stalks. Finely chop the leaves and add half to the tomato and yoghurt mixture. Season the sauce with salt and pepper cover, and chill.

Brush the potatoes under running water, then dry them, and cut into quarters without peeling them.

Peel the shallots and cut lengthwise into quarters. Heat the butter in a large frying pan, then add the potatoes and the shallots. Sprinkle over the remaining spices.

Stir-fry over a medium heat for 10 minutes, then reduce the heat. Continue cooking for another 20 minutes, turning occasionally. Season the potatoes with salt and pepper. Sprinkle over the remaining herbs and serve with the tomato yoghurt.

Serves 2:
1 tsp ground coriander
1 tsp ground cumin
$1/4$ tsp ground cardamom
$1/2$ tsp ground ginger
pinch each of ground paprika, cinnamon, and turmeric
generous pinch of ground nutmeg
2 tomatoes
150 g (5 oz) whole milk yoghurt
5 sprigs of coriander (cilantro)
salt, pepper
500 g (18 oz) waxy potatoes
4 shallots
1 tbsp clarified butter

PER PORTION: 280 kcal • 8 g protein • 11 g fat • 38 g carbohydrate

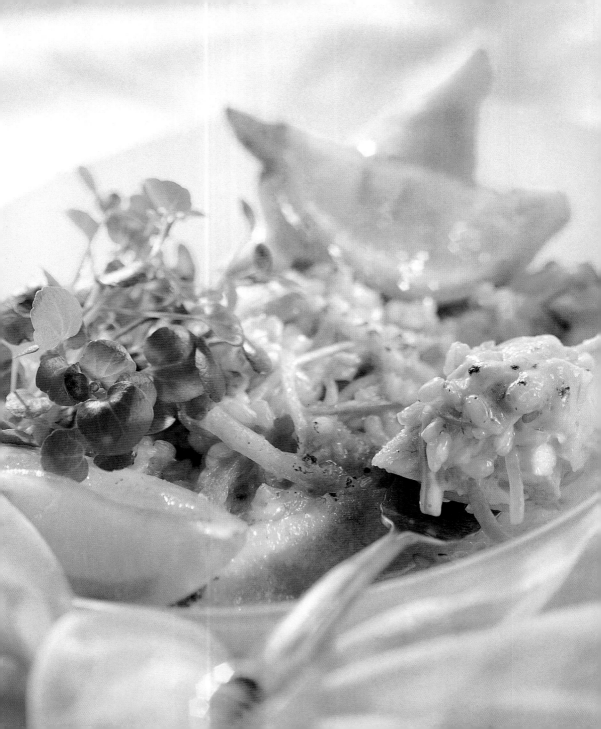

Halibut with a rice and vegetable crust

with plenty of easily digestible protein and fibre

Cook the rice according to the packet instructions. Preheat the oven to 200 °C/400 °F. Rinse the fish under cold water, then dry with paper towels.

Season with salt and pepper, and sprinkle over the lemon juice. Oil the inside of a shallow heatproof dish.

Wash the leek and the carrot. Trim the leek and peel the carrot, then slice both into julienne strips, or dice. Melt the butter in a small pan and braise the vegetables for 2 minutes, then season with salt and pepper.

Drain the rice. Loosely combine the vegetables with the rice, parsley, and Emmental.

Place the halibut steaks in the dish and top with the rice and vegetable mixture.

Bake the fish in the middle of the oven for 20–25 minutes until the topping is crusty. Garnish with the lemon slices and herbs, and serve.

Serves 2:
50 g (scant 2 oz) unpolished white rice
2 halibut steaks
salt
white pepper
1 tbsp lemon juice
oil for the dish
1/2 leek
1 carrot
1/2 tbsp butter
1 tbsp chopped parsley
2 tbsp freshly grated Emmental
4 thin slices of lemon
watercress or parsley leaves

PER PORTION: 520 kcal • 10 g protein • 14 g fat • 50 g carbohydrate

Herb mackerel
with high quality fatty acids and essential minerals
in foil

Preheat the oven to 175 °C/350 °F. Wash the mackerel inside and out, and pat dry with paper towels. Season all over with salt, pepper, and lemon juice, and sprinkle over the herbs.

Serves 2:
2 prepared mackerel
salt
white pepper
2 tsp lemon juice
3 tbsp freshly chopped herbs
150 g (5 oz) low-fat quark
4 tbsp milk
2 tbsp creamy horseradish
1 tbsp capers
1–2 tsp sweet mustard
2–3 tbsp cress

Loosely wrap the mackerel in foil, and place side by side on a baking sheet. Bake in the middle of the oven for 20 minutes.

Meanwhile, beat together the quark with the milk and the horseradish. Finely chop the capers and add. Season with mustard, salt, and pepper. Wash the cress, shake dry, and combine loosely with the horseradish and caper cream.

Serve the horseradish and caper cream with the herb mackerel. Boiled potatoes or a strong rye bread go well with this dish.

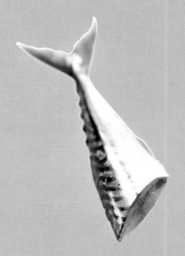

Mackerel

Mackerel is a fish for fitness; it contains large amounts of potassium, iodine, niacin (which is good for the nerves), vitamins D, B_6, B_{12}, high quality amino acids, and omega-3 fatty acids which are a turbo boost for the mood, and provide plenty of power.

PER PORTION:
470 kcal
47 g protein
30 g fat
4 g carbohydrate

power

Oven-baked

a boost for the senses

tuna

Rinse the fish under cold water, then pat dry with paper towels. Sprinkle over the lemon juice and 1 tablespoon of the anise brandy, then chill. Preheat the oven to 225 °C/430 °F. Wash and trim the fennel, then halve, and cut into thin slices. Reserve the green tips.

Peel and finely chop the shallot. Brush the inside of an ovenproof dish with oil. Place the fennel, shallot, and oregano in the dish, and season with salt and pepper. Drizzle over the remaining oil, then pour over the stock and the remaining anise brandy.

Braise the fennel in the middle of the oven for 15 minutes, stirring once. Meanwhile, wash the tomatoes, remove the stalks, and chop the flesh. Season the fish with salt and pepper, and place on the fennel. Top with the chopped tomatoes. Dot with the butter and bake for about 15 minutes. Chop the fennel greens and sprinkle over the fish. This goes well with a crusty baguette, or mashed potatoes.

Serves 2:

2 tuna steaks

1 tbsp lemon juice

4 tbsp anise brandy

350 g (12 oz) small fennel bulbs

1 shallot

2 tsp olive oil

2 sprigs of oregano

salt

black pepper

150 ml (5 fl oz) vegetable stock

3 tomatoes

1 tbsp butter

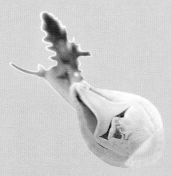

Fennel

Fennel is highly beneficial to both body and spirit. It contains a generous amount of calcium, which is essential to nerves and brain. Iron is needed to ensure a supply of oxygen to the muscles and brain; the essential oils soothe and relax.

PER PORTION:

690 kcal

49 g protein

40 g fat

20 g carbohydrate

Fish soup

exotic and hearty – and filling

with curry

Serves 2:

1 small courgette (zucchini)
2 small red bell peppers
2 tbsp oil
250 g (9 oz) waxy potatoes
1 shallot
1 clove of garlic
2 tbsp grated coconut
1–2 tsp curry powder
500 ml (18 fl oz) vegetable stock
400 ml (14 fl oz) fish stock
(ready made)
salt
200 g (7 oz) perch fillet
4 medium-sized shrimps, peeled
fresh dill tips

Wash, trim, and finely chop the courgette. Halve the bell peppers and remove the seeds and pith. Wash the halves, then finely chop. Heat 1 tablespoon of oil in a pan and sauté the vegetables for 1 minute. Remove, cover, and set aside. Wash, peel, and chop the potatoes. Peel and finely chop the shallot and garlic.

Heat the remaining oil in the pan and sauté the potatoes, shallot, and garlic. Add the grated coconut and the curry powder, and cook briefly. Pour over the stock, then cover and simmer gently for 10 minutes. Add the reserved vegetables, the fish stock, and a little salt. Cover and simmer gently over a low heat for 5 minutes.

Dry the fish and the shrimp with paper towels. Cut the fish into bite-sized pieces. Remove about a quarter of the vegetables from the stock and purée. Add the purée, the fish pieces, and the shrimps to the stock. Cover and cook the fish for about 4 minutes. Season the soup to taste and garnish with dill tips to serve.

power

PER PORTION: 390 kcal • 31 g protein • 17 g fat • 27 g carbohydrate

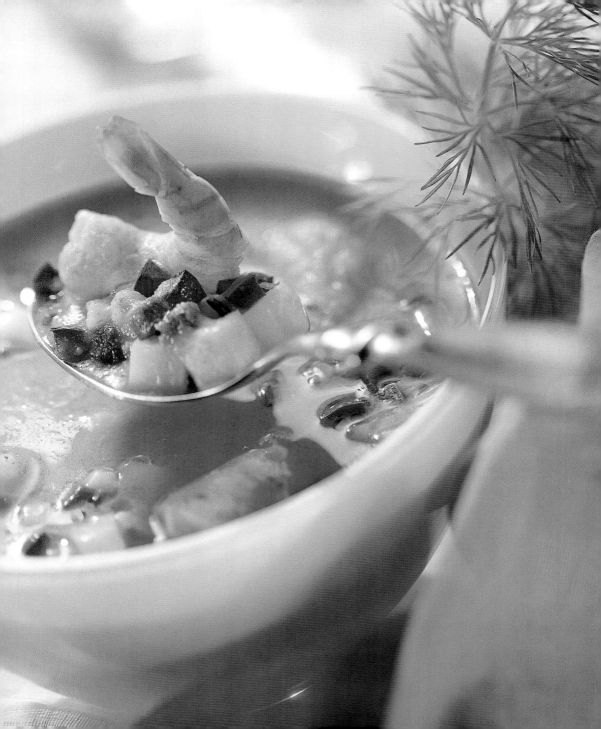

Lamb kebabs
full of protein and carbohydrates
with sesame rice

Cut a cross in the tomatoes and dip in boiling water for a few seconds. Skin, de-seed, and remove the stalks. Finely chop the flesh and sauté in 2 teaspoons of oil until translucent. Add tomatoes, salt, pepper, and maple syrup. Cover and simmer gently for 20 minutes.

Cook the rice according to the packet instructions. Cut the meat into cubes. Halve the bell pepper, then trim, wash, and cut into chunks. Thread the meat and the pepper alternately onto the skewers.

Heat the remaining oil. Fry the kebabs for about 15 minutes, then season with salt and pepper. Dry-fry the sesame seeds and add to the rice. Add the capers to the tomato sauce and season to taste.

Serves 2:
500 g (18 oz) ripe tomatoes
1 small onion
1 clove of garlic
1 ½ tbsp olive oil
salt
black pepper
1 tsp maple syrup
150 g (5 oz) long-grain rice
300 g (10 oz) lamb shoulder
wooden skewers
1 yellow bell pepper
2 tbsp sesame seeds
1 tbsp capers

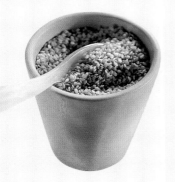

Sesame seeds

They help keep us fit and young. They contain calcium, selenium, silicic acid, and lecithin. Lecithin is essential for nerve function. Choline is an important component in the neurotransmitter acetylcholine, which looks after our nerves, brain, and hormones.

PER PORTION:

585 kcal

41 g protein

15 g fat

71 g carbohydrate

power

Honey-marinated

with courgettes and sun-dried tomatoes

rump steaks

Combine the olive oil, thyme, honey, and pepper. Peel and crush the garlic, and add to the marinade. Dry the steaks with paper towels and brush with the marinade. Cover and leave in the marinade to absorb for 2 hours.

Drain the tomatoes in a strainer, reserving the oil. Wash and trim the courgettes, then cut them in half lengthwise. Slice the courgettes and cut the tomatoes into strips.

Remove the steaks from the marinade and drain. Flash-fry for about 2 minutes on each side in a nonstick frying pan, then gradually add the remaining marinade. Season the steaks with salt, remove from the frying pan, and keep warm.

Add the courgette slices, tomatoes, and tomato oil to the frying pan, and stir for 3 minutes. Season the vegetables with salt, pepper, sugar, and vinegar. Serve the courgette mixture with the steaks.

Serves 2:
2 tbsp olive oil
$1/2$ tsp dried thyme
2 tsp acacia honey
black pepper
1 clove of garlic
2 rump steaks (about 150 g/5 oz each)
50 g (scant 2 oz) sun-dried tomatoes in oil
300 g (10 oz) courgettes (zucchini)
salt
pinch of sugar
1–2 tbsp balsamic vinegar

PER PORTION: 585 kcal • 41 g protein • 15 g fat • 71 g carbohydrate

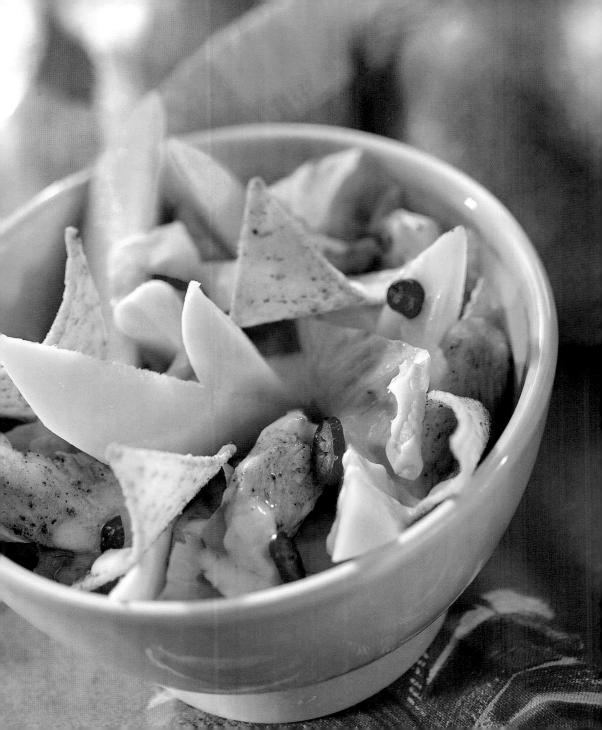

Chilli chicken

a light and fruity recipe from South America

with a mango dip

Peel the mango and cut the flesh from the pit in thick strips. Slice the mango flesh and sprinkle with lemon juice. To make the dip, purée one third of the mango strips with the yoghurt. Wash and shake dry the salad leaves, and tear into bite-sized pieces. Cut open the chilli and slice into thin rings. Dry the chicken with paper towels and cut into strips. Heat the oil in a nonstick frying pan and fry the chicken strips with the chilli until the meat is golden on all sides. Season with salt. Arrange the chilli chicken, salad leaves, and mango strips on plates, and pour over the mango dip. Serve with the tortilla chips.

Serves 2:

1 ripe mango
2 tbsp lemon juice
50 g (scant 2 oz) whole milk yoghurt
4 leaves of lollo rosso
1 red chilli pepper
250 g (9 oz) chicken breasts
2 tbsp oil
salt
50 g (scant 2 oz) tortilla chips

Revive the spirits

Chicken is low fat and easy to digest, and it contains a wealth of vitamins, minerals, and high quality amino acids that are needed to make our body's "messengers" or neurotransmitters. This combination gives us energy, motivation, and revives our spirits.

PER PORTION:

395 kcal

32 g protein

17 g fat

27 g carbohydrate

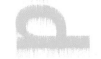

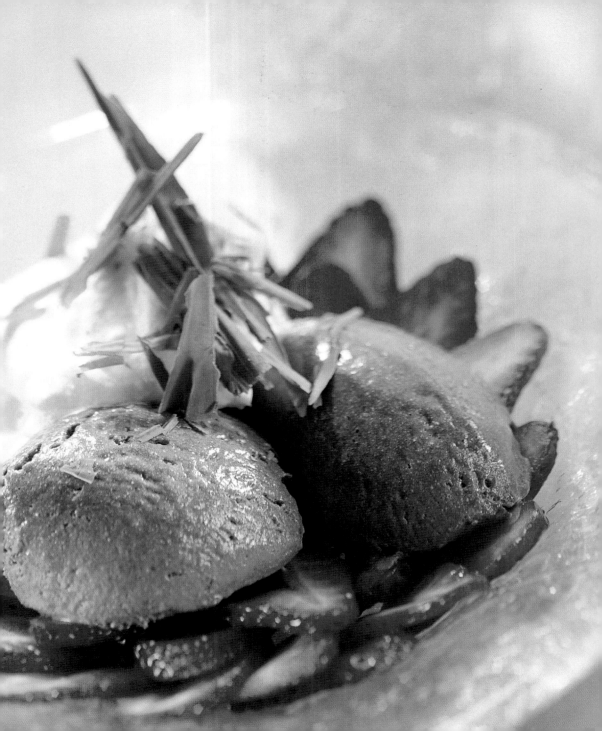

Chocolate
seasoned with cardamom and coffee liqueur
mousse

Break 90 g/3 ¹/₄ oz of the chocolate into pieces and melt in a bowl over lukewarm water, then leave to cool. Meanwhile, dissolve the espresso granules in 2 tablespoons of hot water. Add the coffee liqueur and the cardamom.

Separate the egg. Beat the egg white until stiff, then whip the cream. Combine the egg yolk with the icing sugar, vanilla extract, and 1 tablespoon of lukewarm water, and stir until the sugar has completely dissolved.

Gradually add the espresso and cardamom mixture and the lukewarm chocolate to the creamed egg mixture. Then fold in the cream and finally the beaten egg white.

Divide the mousse between 2 dessert dishes, cover, and chill for at least 2 hours or overnight. Use a paring knife or vegetable peeler to flake the remaining chocolate and sprinkle over the mousse. Garnish with fresh berries such as strawberries, if liked.

Serves 2:
100 g (3 ¹/₂ oz) bitter chocolate
2 tsp espresso granules (or use instant coffee)
2 tbsp coffee liqueur
¹/₂ tsp ground cardamom
1 very fresh egg
75 g (scant 3 oz) whipping cream
1 tbsp icing (confectioners') sugar
¹/₂ tsp vanilla extract

It's got to be right

We all know that chocolate is an ideal remedy if we are feeling tense or upset, but the darker, the better. The higher the cocoa content, and the lower the sugar content, the better it is for us. It's not the amount that helps; eat it in moderation and enjoy it.

PER PORTION:

455 kcal

7 g protein

30 g fat

39 g carbohydrate

power

Mascarpone

with Italian almond biscuits

and cherry cup

Dry-fry the flaked almonds in a small frying pan until golden. Remove immediately and leave to cool. Beat the Mascarpone, vanilla, sugar, and milk in a bowl until creamy, then cover and chill in the refrigerator.

Wash the cherries, then pat dry carefully. Remove the stalks and the pits. Roughly crush the biscuits with the blade of a knife, then sprinkle over the sherry. Layer the Mascarpone cream, crushed biscuits, and the cherries loosely in 2 tall glasses. Sprinkle over the flaked almonds and serve.

Serves 2:
2 tbsp flaked almonds
200 g (7 oz) Mascarpone
pinch of ground vanilla
2 tbsp sugar
60 ml (2 fl oz) milk
200 g (7 oz) sweet cherries
50 g (scant 2 oz) Amaretti
(Italian almond biscuits)
2 tbsp cream sherry

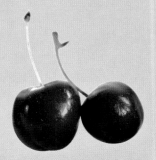

Cherries

Cherries contain a wide range of vitamins, minerals and bioactive plant compounds. The darker the colour of the fruit, the riper and more aromatic they are.

PER PORTION:
735 kcal
9 g protein
59 g fat
37 g carbohydrate

power

Wild honey

refreshing and revitalizing

parfait

Bring a hand's width of water to a boil in a shallow pan. In a heat-resistant bowl, beat together the egg yolks, honey, vanilla, and ground ginger until creamy. Place the bowl in the hot (but no longer boiling) water, and beat with a balloon whisk until the mixture thickens. Remove from the water and continue beating until cool.

Whip the cream until stiff. Fold the whipped cream into the honey mixture, then the yoghurt. Divide the parfait between 2 moulds or cups, cover, and freeze for at least 3 hours. About 20 minutes before serving, remove the parfait from the freezer. Pick over the berries, and wash and pat dry the strawberries if using. Tip the parfait onto flat plates, surround with the berries, and dust with icing sugar.

Serves 2:
2 egg yolks
40 g (1 ¹/₂ oz) honey
¹/₂ tsp vanilla extract
generous pinch of ground ginger
75 g (scant 3 oz) whipping cream
50 g (scant 2 oz) yoghurt (1.5% fat)
250 g (9 oz) wild strawberries or raspberries
icing (confectioners') sugar

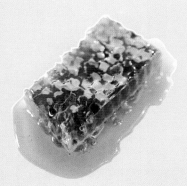

Honey

Honey has a wide spectrum of effects. Its constituent chromium promotes the energy-giving assimilation of glucose in the brain. Acetylcholine speeds up the transmission of signals between the nerve cells, and its gentle consistency soothes the nervous system by releasing calming reflexes via the sensory cells.

PER PORTION:

335 kcal

7 g protein

19 g fat

35 g carbohydrate

power

Figs and
cinnamon surprise

relaxing aroma

Peel the orange and cut out the segments. Place 3 segments in a strainer
and press with a fork to obtain 4 tablespoons of juice. Gently wash the

Serves 2:
1 small orange
3 ripe figs
1 egg yolk
1 tbsp icing (confectioners')
sugar
generous pinch of ground
cinnamon
8 tbsp milk

figs, then pat them dry and cut them into slices.
Place the slices in a bowl and sprinkle 2 tablespoons
of orange juice over them. Cover and set aside.
Bring a hand's width of water to a boil. In a heat-
resistant bowl, beat together the egg yolk, icing
sugar, cinnamon, and the remaining orange juice
with a balloon whisk. Place the bowl in the hot (but
no longer boiling) water and add the milk. Beat

thoroughly with the whisk until you have a creamy foam.

Arrange the figs and the cinnamon foam on plates and serve immediately.

Figs must be ripe

Make sure that you buy figs which are really ripe,
because they are the ones with the unmistakable
aroma and wonderful flavour. Figs taste best slightly
chilled. Peel them if you don't like the skin.

PER PORTION:

135 kcal

4 g protein

5 g fat

17 g carbohydrate

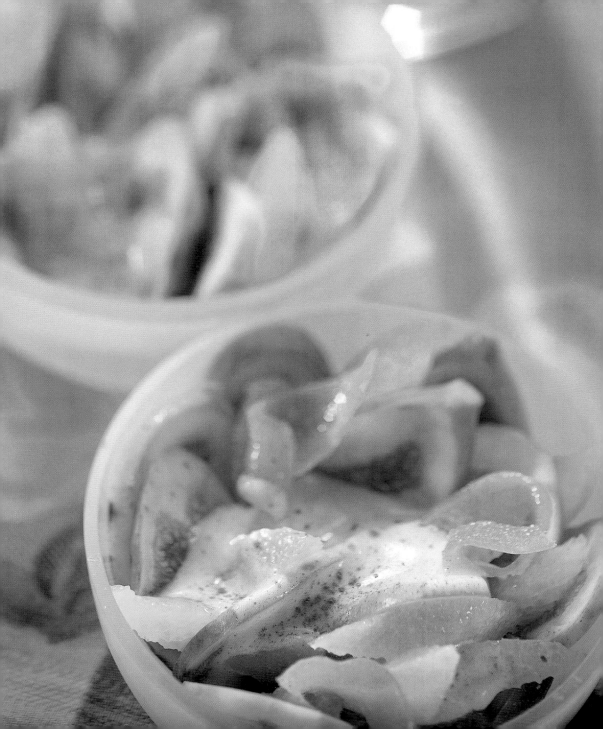

Pineapple and
with lime juice and sesame croquant
papaya salad

Serves 2: • 2 tbsp sesame seeds • 2 tbsp sugar • 1 tsp oil • $1/2$ a baby pineapple • 1 kiwi • 1 small ripe papaya • 2 tbsp lime juice • pinch of ground vanilla

Dry-fry the sesame seeds with the sugar until golden. Pour onto oiled aluminium foil and leave to cool. Peel the pineapple, slice in half lengthwise, and then cut into pieces. Peel the kiwi and the papaya. Cut the papaya into half lengthwise and remove the seeds. Cut both into slices. Combine the lime juice and the vanilla, and coat the fruit in the liquid. Break the caramelized seeds into small pieces and sprinkle over the salad.

PER PORTION: 165 kcal • 2 g protein • 5 g fat • 39 g carbohydrate

Dates on
best chilled
mint quark

Serves 2: • 2 sprigs of mint • 1 tbsp sugar • $1/2$ tsp vanilla sugar • 1 tbsp chopped hazelnuts • 2 tbsp milk • 250 g quark (0.2% fat) • 2 tbsp lemon juice • 8 fresh dates

Wash the mint and shake it dry. Pull the leaves from the stalks and roughly chop. Combine the mint, sugar, vanilla sugar and nuts, and grind well in an electric grinder. Combine this mixture with the milk and the quark, and adjust the flavour with lemon juice. Wash the dates, then dry them and remove the pits. Cut the dates into strips lengthwise. Arrange decoratively on the quark.

PER PORTION: 270 kcal • 19 g protein • 4 g fat • 42 g carbohydrate

Apricot
decorated with pistachios
quark gratin

Preheat the oven to 220 °C/430 °F. Wash the apricots, dry them well, then cut them in half and remove the pits. Cut the fruit into thick slices and sprinkle with the apricot liqueur.

Separate the egg and beat the white until stiff. Combine the egg yolk with the icing sugar, vanilla sugar, and quark, and beat until smooth. Fold the beaten egg white into the quark mixture.

Brush the insides of 2 shallow heatproof dishes with butter. Divide the quark mixture between the dishes and arrange the apricot slices on top.

Bake the gratin in the middle of the oven for 10 minutes. Then increase the heat to 250 °C/500 °F, and bake for another 5 minutes until the top turns golden.

Decorate with the pistachios, and serve warm.

Serves 2:
- 250 g (9 oz) apricots
- 1 tbsp apricot liqueur
- 1 egg
- 1 tbsp icing (confectioners') sugar
- 1/2 tsp vanilla sugar
- 125 g (4 oz) low-fat quark
- 1/2 tsp soft butter
- 1 tbsp chopped pistachios

Infinitely variable
You can use any fruit that happens to be in season or that takes your fancy for this recipe. Bananas, figs, pineapple, oranges, berries, and cherries are all excellent alternatives. You can, of course, also use any combination of fruit.

PER PORTION:

200 kcal

14 g protein

6 g fat

21 g carbohydrate

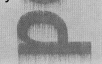

Index

Mood Food

* Abbreviations

tsp = teaspoon
tbsp = tablespoon
kcal = kilocalories

Nutritional analyses in each recipe refer to the metric measurements.

Most of the ingredients required for the recipes in this book are available from supermarkets, delicatessens and health food stores. For more information, contact the following importers of organic produce:-
The Organic Food Company, Unit 2, Blacknest Industrial Estate, Blacknest Road, Alton GU34 4PX; (T) 01420 520530 (F) 01420 23985
Windmill Organics, 66 Meadow Close, London SW20 9JD
(T) 0208 395 9749 (F) 0208 286 4732

Fermented wheat juice is produced in Germany by Kanne Brottrunk GMBH
(T) 00 49 2592 97400 (F) 00 49 2592 61370

Further information on German food importers is available from The Central Marketing Organisation (T) 0208 944 0484
(F) 0208 944 0441

First published in the UK by
Gaia Books Ltd, 20 High Street,
Stroud, GL5 1AZ

Registered at 66 Charlotte St,
London W1P 1LR
Originally published under the title
Rezepte für gute Laune

Nutrition advisor: Angela Dowden

Reproduction: MRM Graphics Ltd,
Winslow, UK.
Printed in Singapore by Imago

ISBN 1 85675 161 9

A catalogue record for this book is available in
the British Library

10 9 8 7 6 5 4 3 2 1

Caution
The techniques and recipes in this book
are to be used at the reader's sole
discretion and risk.
Always consult a doctor if you are in doubt
about a medical condition.

Marlisa Szwillus Studied ecotrophology, and
then joined the editorial staff of a renowned
woman's magazine. For many years she ran the
cookery department of Europe's leading food
magazine. Since 1993 she has been a freelance
food journalist and writer in Munich. She is a
member of the Food Editors Club Deutschland,
and as an expert in her field always combines
healthy eating with culinary pleasure.

Photographs: FoodPhotography Eising, Munich

Susie M. and **Pete Eising** have studios in
Munich and Kennebunkport, Maine/USA.
They studied at the Munich Academy of
Photography, where they established their
own studio for food photography in 1991.

Food styling:
Monika Schuster

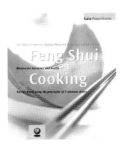

Feng Shui Cooking
Recipes for harmony and
health
Fahrnow, Fahrnow and Sator
£4.99
ISBN 1 85675 146 5
More energy and wellbeing
from recipes that balance
your food.

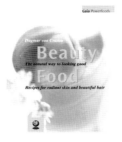

Beauty Food
The natural way to looking
good
Dagmar von Cramm
£4.99
ISBN 1 85675 141 4
Natural beauty for skin and
hair - eating routines for a
fabulous complexion.

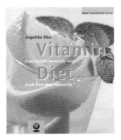

Vitamin Diet
Lose weight naturally with
fresh fruit and vegetables
Angelika Ilies
£4.99
ISBN 1 85675 145 7
All the benefits of eating fresh
fruit and vegetables plus a
natural way to weight loss.

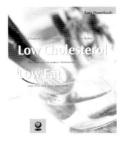

Low Cholesterol - Low Fat
The easy way to reduce
cholesterol, stay slim and
enjoy your food
Döpp, Willrich and Rebbe
£4.99
ISBN 1 85675 166 X
Stay fit, slim and healthy
with easy-to-prepare
gourmet feasts.

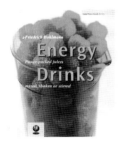

Energy Drinks
Power-packed juices, mixed,
shaken or stirred
Friedrich Bohlmann
£4.99
ISBN 1 85675 140 6
Fresh juices packed full of
goodness for vitality and
health.

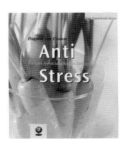

Anti Stress
Recipes for acid-alkaline
balance
Dagmar von Cramm
£4.99
ISBN 1 85675 155 4
A balanced diet to reduce
stress levels, maximise
immunity and help you
keep fit.

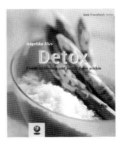

Detox
Foods to cleanse and purify
from within
Angelika Ilies
£4.99
ISBN 1 85675 150 3
Detoxify your body as part of
your daily routine by eating
nutritional foods that have
cleansing properties.

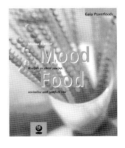

Mood Food
Recipes to cheer you up,
revitalize and comfort you
Marlisa Szwillus
£4.99
ISBN 1 85675 161 9
The best soul comforters,
the quickest revitalizers
and the most satisfying
stress busters.

To order the books featured on this page call 01453 752985, fax 01453 752987 with your credit/debit card details, or
send a cheque made payable to Gaia Books to Gaia Books Ltd., 20 High Street, Stroud, Glos., GL5 1AZ.
e-mail: gaiapub@dircon.co.uk or visit our website www.gaiabooks.co.uk

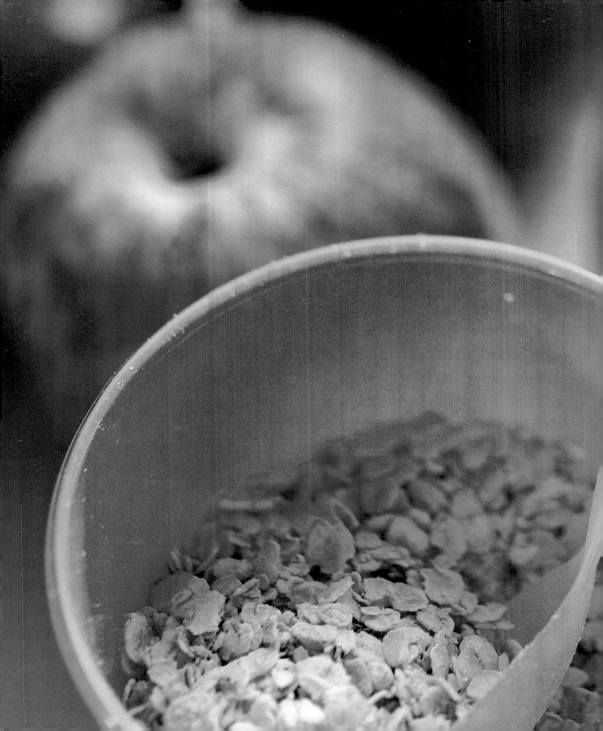